GW00645031

Fitness is not owned by anyone.
It is rented and the rent is due Every Damn Day.
For more tools and resources to help you to get to
a healthy weight and stay there, visit us at:
EveryDamnDayFitness.net

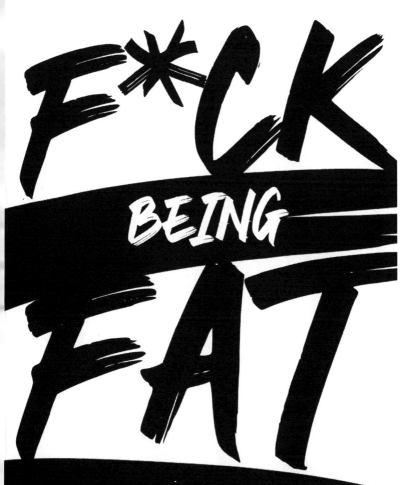

F*CK

BEING

EAT

SOLVE YOUR WEIGHT PROBLEM ONCE AND FOR
ALL WITH **MATH** AND **WILLPOWER**

ALAN ROBERTS

Ordering Information:

Insurgent Publishing books are available at special discounts for bulk purchases for sales promotions or corporate use. Special editions, including personalized covers, excerpts of existing books, or books with corporate logos, can be created in large quantities upon request. For more information, please contact the publisher by email at admin@insurgentpublishing.com.

Although every precaution has been taken to verify the accuracy of the information contained herein, the author and publisher assume no responsibility for any errors or omissions. No liability is assumed for damages that may result from the use of information contained within.

ISBN: 978-1-940715-11-7

Printed in the United States of America
10 9 8 7 6 5 4 3 2 1

DEDICATION

This book, along with everything else I do, is dedicated to my loving wife. She brought love and life to what was just once an existence.

Serenity in the Midst of Chaos.

CONTENTS

PREFACE

BEFORE ANOTHER WORD IS read, please understand that this book is written in my own words. How I talk. How I explain it to my clients and people that come to me for advice on how to lose weight. There will be some colorful language, and, by that, I do certainly mean that there will be words used that some consider profane in nature. So, if you are a precious little snowflake whose eyes cannot possibly read the word "fuck"... I apologize for you reading it this one time, but maybe the rest of this book, and the knowledge within, is simply not for you. If you are not so dainty; if simple letters put together in words that some may consider offensive do NOT offend you, please read on.

First, this will not be some high brow, scientifically documented paper. If you feel the need to check up on what I am stating, please feel free to do so. However, for the fucking record, this book is written as my opinion. Take it how you like. While there are hard FACTS about the nature of food, the calories contained within, and the methods that I used to lose weight myself (the same ones I continue to use to help my clients lose weight), this will not be another book full of pseudoscience (or even actual science) shit. Most of those types of books are designed to confuse the reader and keep them from attaining any type of knowledge (outside leaving them with the generalized idea that they need to buy the next book from the author). This will likely be my one and only book on losing weight, because I do not plan on letting myself get to the stage where I'll ever need to lose weight of that nature again. Once again, this is about how I did it, and how I use the knowledge and tools gained from my personal experience to help others that come to me. Once you understand the MATH, it's as simple as applying WILLPOWER to hit the numbers. That is it.

SOME BACKGROUND

BEFORE I GO INTO the math associated with weight loss (and way before we get into the willpower needed to apply that math effectively), I thought I would give a little background, the goal being to help you understand what I'm saying by providing you a frame of reference for my insights. First, I have been lifting weights and working out for over 30 years. 30 years! And until recently, the only other times I have been sub 15% body fat was when I was a teenager who ran track year-round. This was when I was in my early 20s, when I was very active, and before the isles of all our grocery stores were laden with foods artificially pumped full of extra sodium, fats, and sugars. Remember: If it is labeled low fat, chances are, it is high in sugar and sodium. If it is labeled low sugar, then it is normally pumped full of fat and sodium. Sadly, it just is how it fucking is in our world today. Sugar-filled drinks that our society markets toward the children in our country literally have their own FULL ISLE in most grocery stores, including the "healthy" ones such as Whole Foods and Trader Joe's. Anyway, I digress.

Once, in my early 20s and out on my own, I was, of course, buying my own groceries and not making the best choices. I was, by this time, enamored with lifting weights and changing the 150-pound frame that I graduated high school with only a few years before into what I hoped would look like that of the pro-wrestlers I had grown up watching and admiring. Often eating upwards of 5,000-6,000 calories a day to "gain mass," I would stuff my face full of roughly 1.5 pounds of whatever protein was the cheapest that week. It simply did not matter whether it was steak, chicken, pork, etc. as there was never too much protein in my diet, right? I was always told growing up by the muscle building magazines that to build muscle, I needed to take in protein and A LOT of it. My best educated guess is that I was consuming 250 – 300 grams of protein for roughly 15 years. 1,000 to 1,200 calories in protein alone. Then, of course, I needed to fuel myself. I was a gym bro… I needed to be able to work out for at least 2 hours a day… every fucking day, right? So, for that, I needed a truck full of carbohydrates. It would be nothing for me to, on a daily basis, drink a six-pack of Coca Cola, eat a huge plate of pasta, and eat fried rice from the local cheap-ass Chinese place down the road that would deliver to me. Oh, and beer (yes, beer was part of my training, or that's what I told myself for many years). The calories were useful in gaining mass, and that is what was important, to gain mass. Who cared what kind of mass was built, right? From what I had read, being lean was something anyone could do, whenever they felt like it. All I would need to do when I was ready to have rock-hard, six-pack abs was to add half an hour of cardio a day and eat a few more salads… ok, eat a few salads as there were no fucking salads in my daily consumption at all. There was always time to get lean if I wanted to, except….

Fast forward 20 years, and I have a great life. After many years of personal struggle, which could literally fill another book, the stars seemed to align. Through hard work and the support of an incredible amily, I had success, happiness… all the things that most people wished for when they were younger. The thing was, the time for getting lean never came. While I was not a competitive powerlifter at the time, there was always a desire to be one of the strongest guys in the room. I always craved that. However, it was used as a crutch to keep extra weight on. I would tell myself, "I will lose weight after I squat 500," and then it became, "I will slim down after I squat 600." Even when I would think of slimming down, the idea of taking the 240-pound mass I had attained to under 215 pounds seemed ridiculous in my mind. Why would I want to look that skinny and weak? Plus, I couldn't possibly have that much weight to lose…. could I?

The truth is, I had that much weight to lose, and much more. I was 45 years old and easily at 30%+ body fat. In sitting down and doing the math after going to the doctor, my Lean Body Mass (LBM) was 170 pounds, give or take a pound. My body weight was 243.5 pounds. My body fat percentage was 30.2, and for a mid-40s man, that is life shortening… and I knew it.

I had been in and around the fitness industry for decades, and as I sat there looking at the calculator, I asked myself what I would say if I were one of my clients. I would tell me that I understand that you want to be strong, but don't you want to see your grandkids, that you don't even have yet, get married? I appreciate you love lifting heavy weight, and you think that you need the extra weight to do so, but is that worth developing sleep apnea? I would ask myself if I were one of my own clients, do you not want to hold your wife's hand 30 years from now instead of being a source of pain for her when she thinks about how you died before your time from heart disease or diabetes all because you "wanted" to stay big?

I know those words seem harsh, but honestly, it is the reality. I feel comfortable saying things like this to my clients, even more now, because I have said them to myself.

Bottom line, it was a truly enlightening moment in my life. So, on July 11th, 2017, I set out to change my entire fitness world. I gave myself four months to change my life. I gave myself four months to go from being what is classified as obese for my age and body type, no matter whether it was muscle or fat (a lot more was fat that I would have ever admitted back then), to be at a low-range, body fat level.... lean, athletic…. HEALTHY.

Sitting here now at 187 pounds and at 10% body fat, I remember thinking back then… with only four months to hit my goal (because I set this arbitrary time frame to "challenge" myself and prove it could be done), I needed to plan it out. I knew that while there are many variables in losing body fat, they all fall into one of two things.... MATH and WILLPOWER.

WHAT A DIFFERENCE A YEAR MAKES

THE TWO PICTURES BELOW were taken one year apart in the same fucking shirt. The one on top is from July 2018, and the bottom one from July 2017. While it is customary for the newest one to be on the bottom, fuck that, always put the accomplishment on top!

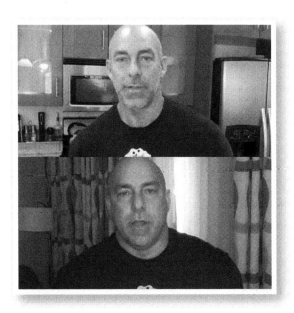

THE MATH

THE MATHEMATICAL EXCUSES

THIS IS NORMALLY THE section of explanation that everyone chooses to ignore for multiple reasons. It seems that it is much easier to listen to that really fit guy or girl on TV or YouTube that has the easy answer; the quick method that asks a person to make one minor change in what, when, or how they eat that will provide them with fast, easy, and sustainable weight loss. People let themselves be sold on the easy, quick fix of magic supplement pills, fat-burning shakes, or "life hacks" that will produce rock-hard, six-pack abs. These things have either incredibly over-exaggerated results or are just flat out bald-faced lies.

The first reason is that people do not want to think about the massive amount of restriction they are going to have to put on themselves. They do not want to "starve" themselves. Our society has rapidly become one in which every meal needs to be thoroughly enjoyable, must taste exactly the way we want it to, and the only meals that that could possibly be repeated in a week are ones of the utmost enjoyment, such as pizza or fast food. If people sat down and calculated how many calories were in the food that they eat, then they would feel bad, so fuck that... ignorance is bliss, and our society has truly become ignorant to the fact that the average person eats like they have a spare body waiting for them.

Secondly, there can often be an incredible and purposeful over-complication of the process needed to lose body fat. I say this is done on purpose because it simply fucking is. Between the various catch phrases and buzz words used to entice and confuse the consumer (who, in this case, could be anyone), the undereducated, serious lifter who is trying to make optimal "gains," the guy that woke up one morning seeing himself in the mirror and realizing he is the poster child for the "dad bod," the person that wants to look good for the beach, to the person that has finally decided to take their doctor seriously about losing weight so they don't die in a few years... the concept of finding a nutritional source to use to lose weight healthily becomes a nearly impossible task that they often either give up on or just pick the person that "sounds the most trustworthy." This over-complication is completely unnecessary, and frankly... bullshit.

Losing weight, specifically body fat, is rather simple in concept. The body needs to burn more calories than it takes in. The math portion of this gets slightly more complicated but is still basic. There are 3,500 calories in a pound of body fat. That is a stated and simple fact. If a person ingests 3,500 more calories than they burn off, they will gain a pound of weight. Again, simple math and facts. Where it gets slightly more complicated is in knowing how many calories the person is taking in and how much they are burning in a day.

AREN'T THERE MORE THAN 3,500 CALORIES IN A POUND OF FAT?

As was discussed earlier, it is often said that there are 3,500 calories in a pound of fat. Before you slam this book down, screaming: "He said it wasn't going to be fucking complicated," just read on for a couple of minutes. One of the many tactics to not fall for is when people try to take away, by either dramatically overstating or minimizing, how many calories are in a pound of body fat. Some "gurus" say it is about half of that, while others say there are 4,100 instead of 3,500 calories in a pound; still others state that calories in vs. calories out don't even matter as there are ways to "trick" your body into being a fat-burning machine. They convince the average dad bod that he can have rock-hard, fucking abs in only a few weeks, and women that they can look like the girls they see on Instagram if they just eat these certain things, or eat at certain times, or whatever else they come up with. These assholes try to over-confuse people to make fuckin money. The truth of the matter is that 3,500 calories being in a pound of body fat is simply a matter of physics.

Kilocalories (from here on in this book are called calories) are a measure of energy. More specifically, it is the amount of energy that is needed to raise 1kg of water 1 degree Celsius. So far, this is just fuckin physics. Now, as will be restated here shortly, when we talk about what food is made up of, there are widely considered to be 9 calories in a gram of pure fat. Notice, I did not say body fat as that is where most of the confusion comes in. Follow along for just a minute.

There are technically 453.59 grams in a pound of any-thing because again... it's fuckin physics. So, 9 calories per gram of pure fat multiplied by 453.59 grams in a pound give us 4,082.31 calories in a pound of PURE FAT. Not body fat... PURE FAT. Just for the record, the 9 calories in a gram of pure fat is also a scientific generalization as there are many studies that show that there are anywhere from 8.5 calories up to 9.7 calories. This would put the calculations for calo-ries in a pound of fat at anywhere between 3,855.5 calories and 4,399.82. However, through exhausting and extensive research, the general scientifically accepted number is 9 per pound of pure fat based on the averages.

Now, I can imagine you sitting there thinking, "This mother-fucker has already said about 10 times that there are

3,500 calories in a pound of fat, but none of these numbers come fuckin' close." Firstly, if you did say that to yourself, maybe you should stop reading this book because my over-use of the word fuck seems to be wearing off on you. I am a fitness personality who is self-employed. I can say "fuck" all I want and can't get fired. You, on the other hand, could be in trouble if you start talking like me. Secondly, and pay attention very carefully, I said 9 calories in PURE FAT. THAT IS PURE FUCKING FAT. I did not say body fat. That is because body fat is not made up entirely of pure fats. Again, there are exhaustive and lengthy studies that go over this, and you are gladly fucking welcome to go look them up if you are one of those assholes that just bought this book (probably pirated it you fuckhead) just to see how many places you can disagree with me. I, however, will not be stopping every two seconds to have the people who purchased this book to specifically find out how I lost 65 pounds of body weight (also known as 26.7% of my body mass in 4 months) look at the citations I picked over the hundreds of other citations that state the same thing. As I stated earlier, this book contains WIDELY ACCEPTED SCIENTIFIC FACTS...and my opinions, of course. Now, back to the fact that body fat is not made up of pure fat, which is why there is the discrepancy that MANY people use to confuse and distort the issue of fat loss. Commonly accepted scientific fact is that there is roughly 87% pure fat in body fat. So if you take the numbers from the pure fat we calculated earlier (453.59 grams in a pound) multiplied respectively by 8.5, 9, and 9.7 (for the low, accepted, and high range of how many calories are in a pound of pure fat) the results are 3,855.5, 4,082.3, and 4,399.8 in total calories. Taking 87% of those numbers (the percentage that indicates how much pure fat is in body fat), we come up with what we more commonly see. Respectively, we see that we in-fuckin-deed have 3,354.3, 3,551.6, and 3,827.8 calories in a pound of body fat. That's why you are told that to burn a pound of body fat, you need to burn 3,500 more calories than you ingest. While it may not be exact, much of this shit won't be either.

This is one of the huge issues that people get caught up in: they will argue over the calories in a pound of body fat, while eating a fat-ass cheeseburger, drinking cola, and smashing fries into their faces. It is an excuse to not look at the big picture. The big picture is that no matter if it is exact or not, it is pretty close, and since, again, as we will fuckin see later, much of this shit is not exact and changes from individual to individual. The big picture is that you NEED to burn more calories than you are taking in, NO FUCKING MATTER

WHAT! If you are one of those people who sat and thought about that in an argumentative fashion:

1. You are a fuckin idiot...
2. It is called reality, deal with it, and...
3. You are still a fuckin idiot.

Now that we have gotten all of that settled, it is time to go on to some of the other portions of the math you need to know (or at least accept to lose weight).

KNOW WHAT IS IN YOUR FOOD

THE FIRST EXERCISES I have my clients start with is to track their food. I have an app of my own that my clients can do this on that also allows me to help them by seeing what choices they are making. Before that, I would always tell people that **if you wanted to reach any physical goal, whether it be to lose weight or gain muscle, you needed to know what you were putting into your body.**

I learned years ago that it is vitally important to understand what your body needs, and in what amounts, to reach your goals. The shock and amazement are always amusing to me when I get the inevitable email or message stating they had no idea how many calories were in one of their favorite foods, or how little protein they were getting while trying to gain muscle mass. I think it used to be much easier when our food was actual fucking food instead of the highly processed items that most people depend upon for their sustenance in our society today. It is truly pathetic that we live in a society where the words "All Natural" can be used as a marketing tool. It is food, it should always be all fucking natural - it's FOOD! However, that is a topic for a different book...

Right now, we are talking about tracking the nutrients that go into your body. These have two basic classifications; Macronutrients and Micronutrients.

Macronutrients, which will be referred to as Macros moving forward in this book, are your basics: protein, fat, and carbohydrates.

Micronutrients are your vitamins, minerals, etc.

Both Macro and Micronutrients are vitally important. One of the excuses I hear all the time from obese people is that they are worried if they diet "too hard" they will not get the needed vitamins and minerals in their diets and could end up being sicker just from dieting. That is when I step in and tell them that they are not "dieting." They are eating the way they need to eat for the rest of their fuckin life. They need to make sure they understand that a diet is a temporary thing. To lose weight and keep it off, *this* is how you fuckin eat now. Only so many calories in a certain time period made up of a certain mix of macro and micronutrients. If YOU are one of the obese people that gets offended when you hear me or others say this, it is simple. You do not need to listen. You can stay eating the way you have, and you can stay obese. You will, of course, die at a much earlier age than those obese people that wake up and realize they need to change their ways. Not to mention, the life you live will be fuckin miserable, as when you get older, it is a near statistical certainty that you will develop a slew of chronic illnesses that are directly linked to obesity. However, the fuckin choice is yours, of course.

PROTEIN

PROTEIN IS THE MACRO that is mostly known as a building block for muscles. It is made up of 20 different types of amino acids and makes up 4 calories per gram when ingested. WAIT!!! Before you close this book or turn away thinking it is going to be another boring manual that discusses all of that, we will not be talking about the 20 different kinds in any depth. Protein is used for many other functions in the body besides building and maintaining muscle, such as for your organs, hair, enzymes, etc. But most of the time when you hear about it, someone is talking about building or maintaining muscle...to the point that it is often abused.

If you've been around a weight room, I am sure you have heard the ridiculous notion that to gain and maintain muscle mass a person needs to ingest 1 gram of protein per pound of body weight. This, in of itself, is idiotic, as it is a blanket statement that doesn't consider a multitude of other factors. To break it down clearly, I will set this scenario. Remember when I was telling you my story about how my Lean Body Mass (LBM) was 170 pounds... well, right now, I weigh 188 pounds.

188 − 170 = 18
(18*100)/188 = 10.1%

So, basically, I am at 10.1% body fat right now. I am pausing to smile at that. Ok, now we can move on. Let's say I have a friend who also has an LBM of 170 pounds, but he is drastically overweight. Let's say he weighs 280 pounds.

280 − 170 = 110
(110*100)/280 = 39.3%

Now, according to the bro-science idiots, I should be ingesting at least 188 grams of protein a day, or I will shrivel up into a wimpy mass and lose all my muscle, and my friend needs to eat at least 280 gram while trying to diet or he will also lose all his muscle. So when he does get to a healthy weight, he would have no muscle mass to speak of. This, of course, is idiot-speak that translates roughly into "I have no idea what the fuck I am talking about." It is simply ridiculous to think that my friend should take in 280 grams of protein a day. At most, my friend needs to take in what I take in, which correlates to an identical LBM number of 170.

My suggestion to all is to take in about 1 gram of protein per pound of lean body mass. Or put simply: YOUR FAT DOES NOT NEED PROTEIN, IT NEEDS TO LEAVE. Why feed your fat when you want it to go away? You do not feed the vermin and raccoons outside your house when you want them to go away. That is how you should treat your fat. The best way to get your LBM number, of course, is by having your doctor do a scan done or, for a little less accurate method, you could visit the gym and have one of the trainers use the caliper method on you. This is rather important for weight loss on two main fronts. First, we do not want to lose muscle mass, and while, as an unfortunate fucking reality, some will be lost, especially when large amounts of fat need to be lost, we want to minimize this as much as possible. And second, while we are losing weight, there is no need to eat the extra calories that would be associated with this piece of fitness mythology that is spread by non-knowing gym bros and protein powder companies. Taking my friend as an example, he should set the goal of taking in 170 grams of protein a day just the same as I would as we have the same LBM. That equates to 680 calories tied up in necessary protein ingestion. If my friend were to listen to the bros at the gym, he would be eating 280 grams of protein even while losing weight. That is 1,120 fucking calories. That is a lot of calories for someone that wants to lose weight, and we haven't even gotten to the other two Macros yet. The idea is to lose weight in a way that is both accommodating to the lifestyle as well as maintainable. A person taking in that number of calories in protein would need to have an enormous energy expenditure to be in a caloric deficit to lose weight since other calories besides just that of the protein will be eaten with the protein.

FATS

THE INGESTION OF FATS has been an interesting topic as of late with the popularization of Ketogenic and Paleo diets as weight loss methods. Before these two fad diets (yes, I called them fads) became popular, eating fat had been seen as eating poison to many. Due to misleading marketing, fat-free diets were all the rage for many years. That fad was just as stupid—in my opinion, of course—as the high-fat diets mentioned before. **The reality is that any diet that restricts any macronutrient is not sustainable in the long term, and, therefore, not something worth using.** That's because the purpose of weight loss is to come to a state of fitness, or general state of wellbeing, in which the body is in equilibrium and operating as efficiently as possible. This simply cannot be done, year after year, by denying the body of any macronutrient over the long haul. Unfortunately, it's a reality in our society. Again, in my opinion, of course.

While there are four basic types of nutritional fats (Saturated, Trans, Monounsaturated, and Polyunsaturated), they can be broken down into two. These are good fats (Monounsaturated and Polyunsaturated) and BAD fats (Saturated and Trans Fats). The good fats tend to be a liquid at room temperature, like vegetable oils, while the bad fats tend to be more of a solid, such as a stick of butter. Now, later in this book, you will remember this and say to yourself, "holy shit, this mother-fucker is telling me to eat bad fats as I eat real butter." I do this to avoid eating overly processed foods, but, as will be seen, this is done in moderation, and only after I have guaranteed my omega 3 and 6 fatty acids, which we will discuss shortly.

For weight loss purposes, keeping fat intake to a minimum is simply in the math. Unlike both carbohydrates and protein that have 4 calories per gram, fat has 9 calories per gram ingested (as we discussed earlier). So, eating high-fat foods is normally problematic when trying to lose body fat for the average person. To be clear, when I say average, I include most of society. Unless you are working out twice a day, have a career that requires serious manual labor daily, or another reason that you are burning an extremely high number of calories due to activity, you are an average person. I know for many, especially many that are avid gym goers, this is a hard concept to accept, but truly a clear majority of people are the average person getting through the day. So, if you are one of those average people like me (even though I own a fitness company to lose body fat), you will want to carefully monitor the amount of fats you put into your body for several reasons. Firstly, a person does not want to cut out fat entirely. Omega 3 and 6 fatty acids are essential to the endocrine system and many bodily functions. Basically, not getting these vital fatty acids can have an adverse effect on the production of hormones, including testosterone, and could lead to lowering of the body's basal metabolic rate making weight loss even harder if not impossible. There is an easy trick to make sure you are getting enough omega 3 and 6 fatty acids, and that is to ingest 2 oz. of walnuts by weight a day...and I hate to have to say this, but ONLY IF YOU ARE NOT ALLERGIC. Sad, that I always must remember that I may be talking to the dumbest mother-fucker to read this book, but it is what it is.

These 2 ounces of walnuts have an estimated 5.1 grams of Omega 3 fatty acids and 21.6 grams of Omega 6 fatty acids. Now, of course, by tracking your food with any of the variety of the apps already highlighted (and that will be discussed later), you may see that you do not need 2 oz of walnuts; maybe just 1. If so, then do so, but make sure you take in the minimums. As the daily recommended amount of Omega 3 and Omega 6 fatty acids are 1.6g and 20g respectively, that makes up an estimated 21.6 grams for 181.6 calories in fat ingestion as a base necessity. As it is impossible to ingest pure Omega 3 and Omega 6 fatty acids, some fats are going to need to be ingested in your nutritional make up.

CARBOHYDRATES

CARBOHYDRATES, OR CARBS AS they will be forever referred to in this book and every gym in the fuckin world, have been both sought after and demonized depending upon which fat or macro exclusive diet trend you adhere to. The category is made up of both simple and complex carbs, and each gram of carbs contains 4 calories. The biggest issue with these calories is that they often leave you craving more calories. Both simple and complex carbs are broken down into sugars in the body that are then housed in the liver until needed. The difference is that complex carbs are considered to be your starchier foods that are also associated with fiber, such as potatoes and rice, and they are not all equal as some are slower to digest than simple carbs, and others have differences in the amount of fiber, density of calories, and other nutrients. Simple carbs digest quickly and often result in feeling hungry shortly after eating. They are digested much quicker as they do not have the associated fiber that complex carbs do. While all carbs, and food for that matter, must be eaten in moderation while you are trying to lose weight, simple carbs are the fuckin devil (they'll leave you hungry again and craving more very fuckin quickly).

If you are someone that has a sweet tooth for snacks and candy and other assorted sugar-laden food products, you will understand this type of craving, as refined sugar is a simple carb. Food items with high sugar content will be discussed later in the Willpower section, as not only should they be avoided due to caloric consumption, they also make it much harder to control food cravings.

Carbs are the big buzz word in the "diet" industry, and this is an issue unto itself. Demonizing one type of macro vs another (or even a particular kind of food) is part of the confusion I was talking about earlier. Personally, I do not like "Macro Exclusive Diets" of any kind as I think they do not build a healthy relationship with food and, for the most part, they are certainly not sustainable for most of the people that use them to lose weight temporarily. For anyone that needs to lose a large amount of weight, it is important to build this healthy relationship with food. Truth be told, and again I do tell hard truths, I have never met a person that is around normal height that weighs over 300 pounds that has a healthy relationship with food. Not fuckin ever!

YOUR BMR

YOUR BASAL METABOLIC RATE, now forever known in the book as BMR because I do not want to fucking type that out every time it is mentioned, is what the sciencey people refer to as the number of calories your body would burn if you did fucking nothing. If you just laid down all day and didn't lift a finger, your BMR is how many calories you would burn. There are multiple different equations that nutrition experts use to calculate this, and they all come up with an acceptably close number to one another (especially considering that the BMR is a very close guestimation of your resting caloric burn, that is then generalized by an activity factor that is truly an educated guess at best, and then compared to calories that are also, at best, guestimated). However, knowing your BMR is an important tool to start you on your weight loss journey. It provides a loose guideline to follow that you can then use to help plan out your nutrition based upon your goals.

HARRIS-BENEDICT BMR FORMULA

THE FORMULA I HAVE chosen to stick with most often is the Harris-Benedict Formula. For those of you picky-ass mother-fuckers who want to backcheck my knowledge or work, please feel free to type harris-benedict+bmr+formula into your search engine search bar. Then pick one of the thousands of articles that come up, as again, I am only discussing things that are commonly accepted as scientific fact. So now that I have pissed off about 10 more people, we can take a look at this method. See below.

For Men:

66.5 + (13.75 * person's weight in kg) + (5.003 * person's height in cm) − (6.755 * person's age)

For Women:

655.1 + (9.563 * person's weight in kg) + (1.850 * person's height in cm) − (4.676 * person's age)

So, using me as an example, currently:

$66.5 + (13.75 * 85.28) + (5.003 * 177.8) − (6.755 * 46)$

Or

$66.5 + 1172.19 + 889.53 − 310.73$

Or

1817.79

If you go to the section in the back of the book, the math for each of these equations is done for you in charts. You simply need to add or subtract as per the equation you are using (either male or female) the numbers that you can get from them. Do not forget to subtract the age number. I have seen that make someone think they have up to 800 more calories estimated they can eat than they actually do.

Basically, the formula states that if I did nothing but lay down every fucking day (long pause with my eyes closed imagining what they would be like then realizing I'd be bored as shit), I would burn 1,817.79 calories. By doing fucking nothing.

Now for the sake of argument, we can see that the older you get, the equation claims you burn fewer calories if you are at rest. So, let us take an average 40-year-old man. We'll call him Hemingway. We will say he is 5'8"/ 68"/ 172.72cm tall. Below, we will show how many calories this 40-year-old male would burn at rest at various weights to show the relative difference.

WEIGHT	200	250	300	400
BMR		1905.5	2209.4	2513.2	3120.9

As you can see above, Hemingway could literally sit on his ass in a sedentary state and burn 2,209.4 calories while weighing 250 pounds. Looking back on our previous math, that would allow Hemingway to eat 160 grams of protein for 640 calories, 100 grams of fat for 900 calories, and another 165 grams of carbohydrates in a day for a total of 2,200 calories, and he'd still be eating under his BMR by 9.4 calories. When eating the right foods, 2,200 calories is filling, nutritious, and frankly doesn't feel like all that much of a fucking restriction.

At 400 pounds, our boy Hemingway is, in my opinion, of course, putting actual effort into either gaining weight or keeping it on. 3,121 calories are either a large amount of nutritious food for a person to eat (especially if they were just sitting on their ass) or a pizza with cheesy bread on the side. That is what it boils down to.

The choices you make about food are the ones that will determine your weight loss. We will get into this in more detail later, but make no fucking mistake, IT IS ABOUT THE FOOD YOU PUT INTO YOUR FUCKING MOUTH. I am sure that the very few smart-ass mother-fuckers left that are still reading this are saying, "but what if he doesn't just lay there? What if he is active?"

To you mother-fuckers, I say, you're right. What if he was active?

Now the Harris-Benedict Formula and the other ones you will find all use similar "activity modifiers" to determine what is called your Total Daily Energy Expenditure, otherwise known as your TDEE. An example of one of the thousands I found is below:

Amount of Activity	BMR Modifying Quotient
Barely Active – You function in your daily life behind a desk and watch tv when you get home almost never getting any other types of physical activity.	1.1
Light Activity – You get 1 to 3 days a week of light activity. 30-minute walks at a slow pace…. Think Walmart shopper.	1.375

Moderately Active – You exercise 3 to 5 days a week. Think gym bro with 5- minute rest between sets of bench and arms.	1.55
Active – You exercise 6 to 7 days a week. You are serious about going to the gym this is a lifestyle for you and you do not fuck around.	1.725
Extremely Active – You exercise 7 days a week with sometimes multiple times a day and or have a seriously physically demanding job. You are a fuckin machine.	1.9

Now we take our boy Hemingway's TDEEs at his different weights.

WEIGHT	200	250	300	400
BMR	1905	2209	2513.2	3120
BARELY	2096	2430	2764.5	3433
LIGHTLY	2620	3037	3455.7	4291
MODERATE	2953	3424	3895.5	5383
ACTIVE	3287	3811	4335.3	5383
EXTREMELY	3620	4197	4775.1	5929

As is clearly seen from the table above, if our boy Hemingway weighed in at 250 pounds and was even moderately active, he would burn over 3,400 calories a day. This brings us to figuring out our deficit.

A final word about these calculations is that they are indeed guestimates. Every person is different, and each person has differences in their BMR due to heredity, environment, and how their body deals with stress. Many of the lying-ass-gurus will use this as a tool to convince people (who are desperate to lose weight, most of the time without actually making any changes to their life) that their methods, supplements, etc. Can help them, and give them an excuse as to why "diets don't work for them." There are even dumb-ass mother-fuckers who try to sell those who don't know better, on how your body type determines the foods you should eat to lose or gain weight. This is all, of course, complete bullshit (in my opinion) as nothing trumps the rules of physics. It is calories ingested vs calories used, and there is no way around that. Do some people burn more than others of their exact age, weight, sex, and height? Of course they do, as every single person is different, but these guestimates give an individual an excellent starting point.

CALORIE DEFICIT: HOW TO FIGURE IT OUT AND HOW TO USE IT

HERE IS THE PART of the book where it becomes obvious why we needed to be clear that there are roughly 3,500 calories in a pound of fat. It is time to figure out how many calories you need to eat to lose weight (based on what you burn). We will refer to this as your **caloric deficit** moving forward to save me from having to type that shit every fuckin time.

For shits and giggles, let us assume that our boy Hemingway weighed in at 250 pounds, so from the chart we have already looked at, we know he has a guestimated BMR of 2,209.4 calories. Let us also assume that our boy Hemingway is LAZY AS FUCK, and while he is not sedentary in bed, he is only lightly active. We can assume his only walking is to and from the parking lot of the grocery store, and sitting up at a desk to do whatever stupid-ass hobby he has. It could be video games, crafting of some kind, who knows, but let us safely assume our boy Hemingway is LAZY. This would give him an activity modifier of 1.1. From the chart above, we can see that gives him a TDEE of 2,430 calories a day. If he eats this every day and has the same activity, he will not lose or gain a pound. It does not matter what he eats. It could be 2,430 calories of jasmine rice or chicken wings. As long as everything else stays the same (including hormone levels, stress hormones, etc.), he will not gain or lose an ounce if he eats these 2,430 calories.

Now, let us say that Hemingway would like to lose some weight. We should fucking hope so because he is an over 40 male who weighs over 250 pounds. That goes downhill quickly, as I can attest to, and, if not caught in time, is life shortening. We will assume that Hemingway wants to lose 50 pounds in this next year. That means he needs to eat 50 pounds worth less than his TDEE for the year. Here is the part that normally makes people say "fuck" to themselves. Since there are approximately 3,500 calories in a pound:

$$3500 * 50 / 365 = 479.45 \text{ rounding up to } 480$$

That is 480 calories a day that he would need to eat less than what he burns, and since he is a lazy fuck and his BMR multiplied by activity modifier is only 2,430 calories, that means that Hemingway can eat 1,950 calories a day every day for the next year and lose 50 pounds.

A good rule to remember is that, in general terms, 96 calories a day is 10 pounds over the course of the year (give or take the variances that occur for each individual and the fact that food labels and their nutritional amounts are also guestimations). 96 calories a day is often the number of calories people take in just by putting cream and sugar in their morning coffee(s). It is that simple.

Now, one thing to remember is that as Hemingway (or anyone) loses weight, their BMR, and thus their TDEE, also gets smaller as they do not weight as much and, therefore, do not burn as many calories through metabolic and activity. This is one thing that obese people face as they lose large amounts of weight. This is also one of the many reasons that diets do not work. A diet temporarily reduces the caloric intake of an individual. A new lifestyle includes eating only a certain variance of calories that support their new weight.

THE MATH OF MY WEIGHT LOSS

How did I determine my caloric intake for losing weight? I was 243.5 pounds at 45 and between 5'9" and 5'10" depending upon the doctor's office I would go to. As I already worked out, 5 to 6 days a week, my activity level was considered active, thus, my TDEE was:

$$66.5 + (13.75 * 110.45) + (5.003 * 177.8) - (6.755 * 46)$$

Or

$$66.5 + 1518.7 + 889.53 - 310.73$$

Or

$$BMR = 2164$$
$$TDEE = 2164 * 1.725$$

Or

$$3732.9$$

Now, because I put a 122-day time limit on myself, I couldn't just lose the 60 pounds by eating in a deficit of 96 * 6 = 576 calories a day as I did not have a whole year to do it in (basically, because I said I would lose the weight in 122 days like an idiot). So, since I had 122 days to lose 60 pounds, I did the math like this:

60 pounds * 3500 calories in a pound

Or

210,000 calories of deficit
210,000 / 122 days

Or

1,721 calories a day of deficit.

Since I had an approximate TDEE of 3,733, I subtracted the 1,721 calories of deficit I needed to lose the weight in the time frame and came up with 2,012 calories a day. I rounded this down just for simplicity to 2,000 calories a day, and that is what I did. I averaged eating approximately 2,000 calories a day every day for 122 days.

Were there days when I ate a little more? Abso-fuckin-lutely there were. But those days were always accounted for. The way I would do this was that if I knew I would go over my calories on Friday taking my wife out to dinner, I would simply eat 1,800 on the Wednesday and Thursday before as well as the Saturday afterward. This way, I could feel comfortable eating 2,600 calories one day of the week. This also allowed me a mental break from the 2,000 calories, which I found very important but will talk about later in the willpower section of the book.

Now, how did I deal with the rapid reduction in my TDEE that came along with the rapid reduction in my weight (often losing 3.5 pounds a week, especially at the beginning)? I did this thing called getting my ass moving. I am not going to make this into an exercise book, or an avenue to sell my workout programs or coaching, but I can tell you that as I got lighter, I became much more active. Once I was motivated and saw the weight coming off, it was easy, as I was excited to see the progress on the scale weekly and, toward the end, in the mirror daily.

While you cannot out-exercise poor eating habits, you can definitely use activity to burn calories along with proper nutrition. The problem is that people are more willing to do exercise, but not the nutrition in most cases. Think about it this way, if you work out for a half an hour, most people burn about 250 to 300 calories or roughly the calories in a 20 oz bottle of soda. Think about that every time you go through a drive-through. Half hour on a treadmill for one large soda from the obesity convenience window.

This is the thing the exercise gurus (the shredded abs in 5 minutes a day mother-fuckers, the 10 minutes to trim bullshitters, and all the other mother-fuckers that are just in it to get your money and show you just enough results to get you to buy the next level of their package) do not want you to realize.

You CANNOT out-exercise eating too much shitty food. You simply fucking can't.

To make matters even worse, most people that need to lose a large amount of weight are not even physically capable of the activity they would need to be able to burn the calories needed to lose that weight. The weight they need to lose to live to old age if they do not change their eating lifestyle. Yes, they may be able to lose 10 to 20 pounds in a certain amount of time by listening to the really pretty mother-fucker with the great abs on YouTube or TV, but doing the minimal amount of exercise a seriously overweight or obese person can do will not negate a large pizza. These gurus know it. That is why they give advice like "eat clean," "eat fewer carbs," "don't eat after 6 pm," and all sorts of other stupid-ass bull-shit that gives no real specifics, knowledge, or information. It just seems like a fuckin side note to the "5 minutes and 5 exercises to no love handles" sales pitch.

That is one of the reasons why I decided to write this book: to put out in VERY simple terms, because I am a very simple man, the math and knowledge that a person needs to be able to at least know what targets they are shooting for when they decide it is time for a change. When they decide to trade in the all the inevitable ailments, pains, and chronic illnesses that come along with being overweight and obese in exchange for an active and happy life (and where they can shop at stores that make clothes for normal sized folk).

THE MATH OF TRACKING YOUR FOOD

I WILL TALK A little bit later about how important it is to track your food. There are some that disagree with me. I even have a very good friend who is widely considered one of the best trainers in the country that does not coach tracking calories, just balanced eating.

The difference between us is who we coach.

My friend coaches almost exclusively athletes. People with large energy expenditures who eat every single day with the intent to burn every calorie.

I, on the other hand, coach mostly overweight to the morbidly obese.

My people simply aren't getting the same type of activity as my friend's clients so that makes a huge difference in how we coach them. My friend's people are also not food addicts, which most of mine are. When a person's relationship with food is bad, they have to track it. However, I am getting off topic for now.

Tracking your food is just like the rest of the math when it comes to activity: how many calories are in a gram of food or macronutrient are all guestimates. They are educated guesses with varying degrees of accuracy, and food tracking apps are no different. The differences lie in their estimations at many levels. As an example, one four-ounce chicken breast will not have the same nutrition as another for a variety of reasons. The two chicken breasts will almost certainly have different hydration levels, so while they both could weigh exactly the same, one could have substantially more water in it than the other. The point is, even estimates are better than nothing.

WILLPOWER

THE HARDEST PART...
HAVING WILLPOWER

THIS IS THE HARDEST part of the book. It's the hardest part of the book because most of it is up to you. **If you cannot develop the willpower to stick to nutritional goals based on long term health, you will never, ever, be healthy.**

Sadly, in our society, I would imagine that about 50% of the people that will read this book will read that last sentence and say, "fuck it." These are the people that are feeding the "quick fix," "eat all the foods you love," "absolutely no hard workouts, and you lose weight" assholes that take advantage of those that either do not know any better or choose to try every other option possible to not have to do the one thing that will actually get them to a healthy weight.

The people that are constantly searching for that one golden, glorious, mother-fucker that has somehow found that one, simple thing that has been missed by ALL of the scientists who have studied nutrition, metabolism, and all the other aspects that go into health related to weight loss, are probably going to throw this book down. They are going to say, "he's a scamming piece of shit" to themselves, and storm off pissed because, basically, I just said they are going to have to do the one thing that they fucking HATE to do...

To those of you that felt that way, get the fuck over it, because the reality is nobody can lose weight for you. You are the one that needs to find the reasons. You are the one that needs to find the self-control to monitor yourself. **You are the one that needs to learn how to tell yourself NO.**

In this section of the book, I am going to try to help you by telling you what I said to myself, my clients, and people in my life who wanted to lose weight. These are things I used to help motivate them to get and stay healthy. I am also going to share strategies that will help you say "no" to yourself (or at least make it easier).

These are not fixes, but they may just help you.

The most important point is this: regardless what strategy or technique you use, whether it's one of the suggestions I give, or it's something you completely make up on your own, you need to use it. You need to apply it to the math we have already gone over, and, from there, develop a plan to get healthy.

If the terms "very overweight" or "obese" apply to you, you need to start today.

Not tomorrow or after the holidays or when your friend starts with you. If you are obese, you are actively shortening your life, and, as said before, making the years you have less enjoyable by wrapping yourself in a self-made prison made of your own body fat.

I know we live in a politically correct culture, and there are even groups such as the "Fat Acceptance Movement" that will try to tell people that they are ok at any size. What medical science, statistics, and, most importantly, *reality*, state, are that while a person can still be a great individual with a loving heart, they are hurting themselves by staying in an obese state. This, again, just like all of the other things I have pointed out, can be seen with one press of an enter key after typing the words "chronic obesity illness" into a search browser.

People telling a fat person that they are healthy at any weight is not only an ignorant dismissal of the truth, I personally believe it is a form of bullshit like no other. Statements like this, frankly, kill people (in my opinion, of course). Believing statements like these shortens lives, takes mothers and fathers away from their kids, and robs grandchildren of ever getting to know their grandparents.

The people that say not to worry about the weight to an obese person are even worse than the money-hungry gurus with the 5-minute abs commercials who profit off the ignorant. At least with the guru, some activity is involved. These people rob an obese or overweight person of the reasons to get healthy, because they love to believe the lie. The lie is: that they do not need to get healthy. That there is literally nothing wrong with them; that a large pizza is normal to eat 5 times a week.

So don't listen to the phonies, charlatans, and scammers. Take ownership of your weight, your life, and your future. Only *you* can. Only *you* can care enough to make the changes in your life that you know need to be made. And that's as good a time as any to get into the WILLPOWER side of the equation...

THE REASONS TO HAVE WILLPOWER

I AM NORMALLY NOT like this, but I really do feel I should give a little bit of a disclaimer with this section. I am going to tell some stories about some of the things I have said to myself and others to make them understand the importance of having the willpower to lose weight and get healthy. If this book is the first thing that has ever exposed you to me, first, holy shit, thank you for making it past all the fucks, bullshits, and mother-fuckers used in the book so far. Please do understand that there will be many more in the pages to come.

Second, I do not sugarcoat shit. I take all sorts of clients in my coaching, both online and in person, but a vast majority of my clients start out very overweight to morbidly obese. This is mainly due to them realizing that while what I say to them can sound very harsh, it comes from a place of wanting them to see what is in store for them, for their loved ones, and for their future (or lack thereof if they do not get healthy). So, just to understand, the stories that are about to be told will not use the person's real name, and I will paraphrase as much as I can to change the story slightly so as not to "out" anyone, but know that the clients that I speak of have all told me that they hope I am able to use their stories to help others decide to fight to escape the prison of fat that comes with obesity.

450

ONE OF MY VERY first online clients is still with me today. When he reached out to me, he had a body weight of 450 lbs, so that is what we will call him in this story: 450.

450 messaged me on social media out of the blue in early October of 2017. I was over halfway through my weight loss and had lost over 40 pounds. He had seen a YouTube video I had done on a popular gaming YouTuber who had undergone gastric bypass surgery. In the video, I stated that treating the food addiction of a morbidly obese person by reducing the size of their stomach was similar to cutting the thumbs off of a drug addict's hands so they couldn't push the plunger of the syringe in. In a vast majority of cases, both the drug addict without thumbs and the food addict with the small stomach, would find a way to feed their addiction, whether it be by finding a new one, or a new way to feed the one they currently had.

This analogy had an effect that I did not predict. Again, for those of you that do not know me outside these pages, I say crazy bullshit all the time. I specialize in taking harsh realities and placing them in front of people and making them look at them. I have used my brand of satirical comedy to point out when I have thought people were doing things without the best interest of their followers at heart, and I have called people serial killers, punk ass bitches, mother-fuckers (really, a term of endearment from me at this stage), and many other things. I have had other people's fans mad to the point that they leave mean comments, send nasty emails, a few death threats here and there, fake accounts in my name, hacking attempts… basically, all the normal things you would imagine someone like me would get.

However, this analogy took things to an entirely new level. The gaming YouTubers' fans went FUCKING CRAZY. Phone calls, death threats, THOUSANDS OF COMMENTS on all my social media. It was fuckin nuts. That shit was truly crazy, but the cool thing was that it resonated with some people. In fact, my first few online clients came from that video. 450 was the first, but there were several others (all morbidly obese) who reached out due to that very video, which made it all worth it.

When he messaged me on Facebook, it read as you would imagine from someone that had felt like he tried to lose weight his entire life but couldn't. He told me of all the diets he had been on. Told me that he knew he was a food addict and that he couldn't say no to pizza. He told me that he was diabetic and worried about losing his legs because that is what happened to his dad who, sadly, could also be named 450. His dad passed away when he was only 50 but had not had his legs below the knees since he was 40.

450 was 36 years old at the time.

I messaged back, and we arranged a video chat. I was absolutely sure that he was going to hate me because, let's face it, telling a person they are addicted to food, and they have to not eat the way they have been, is normally not met with happiness. When we got on the call, I remember thinking, holy fuck, this guy is dying in front of me. His skin color screamed high blood pressure. His skin presented as a person who ate a lot of oily food, and you could look at him and know he poured table salt on everything from how puffy he looked.

We introduced ourselves. I asked him to tell me how I could help him. 450 said he had tried everything, even hypnotherapy. He was on the biggest dose of anti-depressants that he could be on without having a serious adverse effect on his blood pressure, cholesterol, and heart medication. He hated his life, and the only thing that made him feel any better was food.

What I said next stopped him in his tracks: "So because you hate your life, you are committing suicide by food?" I asked him.

I could tell on the video chat that he thought maybe I didn't understand. He said. "no, I said food is the only thing that makes me happy."

From there, I told him very plainly that for him to be able to move forward, he needed to realize that food was *actually* the thing that was making him sad, and it had been his whole life. 450 didn't have any kids. He and his wife had chosen not to because they both came from morbidly obese families and had both lost parents at a young age and didn't want to see that happen to their kids. For both 450 and his wife, their parents' food addictions had scared them so much, they made the active decision to not have kids in fear of them dying young. Food took the thought of children away.

When I said that to him, his face dropped. I then told him that he needed to accept that he was using food to slowly kill himself. He knew it would eventually lead to his early death, and yet, he was still eating a large pizza 3 to 5 days of the week (which is just utterly fuckin insane).

In no way was I trying to be mean to him. He told me later that he knew it, but I was saying things to him that nobody else had. Others had tried to help him cope with his eating habits, they had tried to soft-handedly make it about moderation and exercise.

I told him you can have 2,500 calories a day, and I expect to see a video of you walking at a 2-mph pace (or faster) sent to my phone, 5 days a week, with that day's newspaper visible. I thought for sure he was going to be offended by the "paper from that day" comment, but the mother-fucker literally freaked about the 2,500 calories in a day.

"That will be like torture," he said loudly to me. I asked him would be it more torturous than the doctors cutting off both of his legs in 3 years? He paused.

I added that he could use his father's old wheelchair. Tears rolled down his face as I said, "close your eyes and picture that. Imagine what you would look like in your father's old wheelchair."

More tears as 450 began to sob. He screamed at me, "you don't think I have nightmares about that?" I said, "apparently not enough or this would be a simple conversation. Do you want my help or not? If you do, it's 2,500 calories a day, and when you send me the video clip of you on the treadmill, make sure to send pictures of all the food you have eaten that day and the days you weren't on the treadmill, so I can see your portion sizes."

450 is now 370, and I am very proud of him. He is still in the danger zone, and has a long way to go, but he has also had a tough year family-wise, and I am very proud that he has not relapsed to the scale going back up.

DQ

THE NEXT STORY IS of a client. We will call him DQ. He came to me about a week after 450, and while not quite as badly off, he was a very big man. 6'6" 400 pounds of a big man. On our first video chat, I was a little surprised by him.

"I know I am a food addict," he said immediately after I asked what I could do for him. I was a little shocked but asked him to tell me about it. DQ was a contractor, and a successful one. He ran his own company and did very well for himself. He had 3 kids; the oldest was 8, the youngest was 6 months. He had always been big, but he had put on 50 pounds in the last year as "sympathy weight" for his wife being pregnant with their 3rd child. He said, "I know I am in trouble."

I asked him what the food was that he couldn't say no to. He then told me about how his office was about a 15-minute drive in the mornings and about 1 hour and 15 minutes in the afternoon due to traffic. He said he had always had a sweet tooth, but one day, right after his wife got pregnant, she asked him if he would pick her up some chocolate ice cream from Dairy Queen. He didn't like chocolate, so he picked up a vanilla cone for himself. The next day, on the way home from work, about a mile before he was normally stuck in traffic, he saw a Dairy Queen, he pulled in and got himself a small cup of vanilla ice cream to eat while stuck in traffic.

By the end of her first trimester, he was eating a family-sized vanilla tub in the car every day.

He said he was always big, but was gaining weight faster than he ever remembered because he couldn't say no to pulling in and getting his vanilla ice cream. DQ was fully addicted to DQ. His wife was seriously concerned, as was his doctor. DQ had a home gym and lifted 4 times a week to try to shed the weight, but he kept gaining.

So I said to him that the solution was pretty easy: he needed to stop eating Dairy Queen completely and manage his calories to slightly below what he would have been eating before he started the Dairy Queen binge. He said of course he knew that, but he had to find a way not to. So, the first thing I did was make him install an app so his wife could track his phone by GPS. They also set a phone date to talk while he was on his way home from work. Then, and most importantly, I had him leave an hour earlier to get to work and an hour earlier to get home...and I changed his route.

It was still an hour and fifteen minutes home every day, but he did not pass a single Dairy Queen on the way home.

Things were going well, and then about 3 months in, he stopped checking in with me. I waited a few days and then reached out. He had slipped, literally just like an alcoholic or drug addict, and eaten Dairy Queen every day that week. He said he wanted to reward himself a little. I said — and I fuckin quote — "you have rewarded yourself enough. You do not get a fuckin reward for shit you should do. I want you to imagine your six-month-old daughter 22 years from now. She is in a beautiful white dress at the end of an isle with everyone she knows. She is about to marry the man of her dreams, and it should be the happiest day of her life, but instead, she is crying because all she can think about is that her dad wasn't there to give her away because he couldn't say no to Dairy Queen."

The look on his face on the video chat was of sheer anger. I am sure if we were in the same room, his big ass would have beaten me down - seriously sure. "Close your eyes and picture it! Imagine your daughter crying because Dairy Queen was more important than her!" I said.

The anger turned to pain in his face. I said, "Do you see her? Do you see her crying?" He whimpered slightly and said in a very different voice, "I see her."

I sat for a second and then said, "Good! Remember the white on her dress the next time you treat yourself to your vanilla ice cream."

As of the writing of this book, DQ is now at a lower weight at 310 pounds than he was when his wife got pregnant. He has lost 90 pounds in just about 10 months, and I couldn't be prouder.

These are just a couple of examples of how I coach people. How I help give them a reason to lose weight. The thing is: they already know it. They can already see it in their mind. They are just trying hard to deny it. They do not want to admit it to themselves the harsh truth, but it is already there. That is why I am able to get them to see it so easily. Any obese person KNOWS that they are not healthy. They know that they will not live a full life span, and they damn sure know that they are leading a limited life while they are alive. The reason is there and known. They just need to admit it.

SOME TOOLS AND STRATEGIES

HAVING THE WILLPOWER TO say no to eating more calories than your nutritional plan is, of course, a matter of self-control. However, there are multiple tools at your disposal to make life just a little bit easier, and to make it easier to say "NO" to yourself when it comes to your favorite food. I can personally attest to knowing that resisting a piece of pizza was much easier if I did not feel hungry. I think that is one of the things that fucks with people so much when they go to lose a large amount of weight. The thought that they will be hungry, day after day, after day, and have to deprive themselves of the foods they love.

While it is absolutely true that there will be times that a person will feel hungry when they start on their weight loss journey, that does not mean that they need to suffer needlessly. Below are several of the methods I used and still use today to both restrict my calories and have the utmost satiation that I can have in a day.

HYDRATION AND DRINKING YOUR CALORIES

THERE ARE SEVERAL METHODS that, of course, tie in together, but this one is by far the most important in my opinion. So many people simply do not realize how many calories a day they fucking drink. Earlier, we discussed how removing something as simple as cream and sugar from your morning coffee could lead to 25 to 30 pounds of weight loss in a year.

I have had clients who, when examining their nutritional intake for the first time, had a fuckin epiphany that they were drinking close to 1,000 calories a day. Between gas station soda dispensers, Starbucks' cappuccinos, whole milk, and fruit juices, people ingest calories needlessly that are also normally packed with sugar, possibly causing them to crave more foods later.

If a person is truly serious about their weight loss, they will drink less than 1% of their daily calories a day. So, if you are on a 2,000 calorie a day budget, you will drink less than 20 calories a day.

Taking myself as an example, the first thing I do in a day when I wake up is drink about 20 ounces of water. This not only hydrates me, as I have been sleeping for 5-7 hours and have slightly dehydrated myself just through normal expiration, but it will also fill up my stomach. Very shortly, I will get to how I do not eat breakfast, but even if I did, I would be less inclined to eat a larger breakfast as my stomach is now full of water. I am satiated. I then have a very large BLACK coffee... no fucking cream... no fucking sugar. I normally have a second one, so by the time I have been awake for a few hours, I have drunk about 50 oz of fluids and less than 15 calories.

Compare that to a person who drinks a morning coffee with cream and sugar, plus a glass of orange juice (which is known in the fitness world as sugar water and literally worse than most fucking sodas), and who is at over 300 calories with less fluid, thus less satiation. And that is not even talking about possibly feeling hungry earlier due to ingesting more than 50 grams of sugar before they step out of the fucking door.

I normally suggest to clients that they take in 32 grams of sugar or less in a day if they are at all serious about their weight loss.

Add to all this, I personally find that most people do not pay nearly close enough attention to their hydration, which can lead to a multitude of issues, the least of which being water-poor sleep and water-weight retention.

FASTING

THERE HAS BEEN AN incredible influx of gurus monetizing terms like "intermittent fasting" for the last several years. With claims of increased growth hormone levels, increased fat loss, better sleep, more energy, that it cures diseases, and so many other things that all do have some basis in actual science, gurus have found methods to help people only eat food during a certain window of time. The very popular one is the 16/8 method in which a person eats all their calories within 8 hours and ingests 0 calories for 16 hours.

Personally, I do not give much credit to the boisterous claims that normally come along with the different types of fasting, as in my opinion, the science is far from settled. What I can tell everyone is that skipping a meal allows you to feel fuller at the ones you do eat.

I haven't eaten breakfast except for special occasions for about a year now. I do not miss it... at all. When I wake up at 4 am, I drink my 20 to 30 ounces of water as stated before. Have a large coffee or two and then go about my day until about noon or 1 pm.

During that time, I focus on drinking water every hour or so to get as much hydration early in the day as possible. I make sure I stay hydrated. My stomach stays full, so I am not hungry at all. And I am not drinking a ton of fluids before I go to sleep, which would result in my old ass having to wake up and piss multiple times through the night fucking up my sleep pattern.

Then I have my lunch. Normally, my lunch consists of mostly protein with some fibrous vegetables, such as broccoli or legumes of some kind. I am normally still decently full of water, so this smaller volume meal that normally accounts for about 25% to 33% of my total calories for the day is more than enough to fill me up. Again, leaving me full and not hungry at all. I then go on about my day until about 7 pm when the wife and I enjoy a pretty balanced dinner that is the rest of my 66% to 75% of my total calories for the day. I normally eat the 2 oz of walnuts that I discussed earlier while I am cooking this meal composed of lean protein, vegetables, and a small number of complex carbs. The ratio of the plate is normally one fist-size portion of protein, 2 fists of vegetables, and the inside of my palm-sized portion of carbs.

OMAD

OMAD STANDS FOR ONE Meal A Day. Basically, it is intermittent fasting with the feeding window being the time it takes you to eat your one meal and the rest of the day eating nothing else.

Now before those people that have made it all the way into this book (or skipped to this section to see what I was going to say about this) get their fuckin panties in a wad, I want to add a disclaimer that I think of this method as a temporary fix, one that cannot truly be utilized by most people who are just starting their weight loss journey as it requires a great deal of willpower. It can be a truly effective tool for weight loss for sure, but it is not all that easy for people that are used to feeling full all day long. You will have a portion of the day when you will feel hungry. Straight the fuck up!

I use this method occasionally when I drop my calories very low; when I want to decrease my body fat percentages for merely aesthetic purposes. I do not find that I performed well athletically during these times as most of my workouts were done while fasting. My morning workout is always fasted, so this was no big deal, but my afternoon workouts are normally after my protein meal at lunch. Those workouts DEFINITELY suffered.

The "why" I do this occasionally is simple: I have found that once I cut calories to or below 1,800, that splitting it into 2 meals a day left me hungrier than I liked at night. This has a negative effect on my sleep, and I will get hungry earlier than my set meal times started. So, I just decided that if I was going to be hungry, I might as well only feel it during the fucking day.

The "how" I do it goes pretty much like this. I'd wake up and do my normal daily routine drinking water then coffee and fast until noon. At noon, when I would normally eat, I would get in some type of activity. Usually an "Every Minute on the Minute" workout. Meaning that I would do X amount of pushups, X amount of body weight squats, and X amount of another exercise, every minute at the beginning of the minute, and then catch my breath for the rest of that minute until the timer went off. Since I am never hungry after a fucking cardio session, which this basically is, it would satiate my hunger temporarily. I would, of course, follow this up with rehydration to replace the fluids I'd lost in the workout, and that normally lasts an hour and fills my belly, further satiating my hunger.

The issue is that no matter what, I needed to stop drinking a lot of fluid before around 5 pm or I was going to have to fucking piss all night long, which would also fuck up my sleep. So, from about 5 pm until 7 pm or so, I would be SERIOUSLY FUCKING HUNGRY! Seriously hungry, to the stage that I would get irritable, pissed off easily, and basically not fun to be around. However, at 7, I would eat a meal that consisted of all my calories during the day.

This HUGE meal was almost always the same thing: I would eat my 2 oz of walnuts during the cooking process to start my system off slowly as there hadn't been a single piece of food in my fuckin stomach all day. I then ate almost the same thing every single time. I would have 3 cups of peas, 2 cups of broccoli, 16 oz of riced cauliflower, and about a pound to 20 oz of tuna or salmon depending upon what I needed to get to my protein goal of 160 grams. I would lay the veggies down in a steel pan with a little water. Season them generously and then place the pieces of fish on top putting a lid on them. I would then turn the burner on and wait for the veggies to steam the fish to doneness. I would throw that all into a bowl, season some more (often with mustard, which I absolutely crave when cutting calories) and eat the HUGE MEAL.

Nearly every time, I had to make myself finish the meal as I would be full about 75% through but had to eat the rest as I didn't want to miss my macros. I would be fucking stuffed by the end, but it did allow me to sleep like a fuckin rock every single night.

As I stated, it is not (in my opinion, of course) a way to lose weight while keeping athletic performance. Thus, why I only do it for a week or two at a time. It is, however, a way to cut an extra 300 to 500 calories from my normal cutting protocols to lose an extra pound or two over the course of a week or two.

SELF-SOCIAL MEDIA ACCOUNTABILITY

ONE OF THE TOOLS I have used on myself in the past as well as my clients is to send a picture of everything I do to someone else. I personally used my social media as a method to hold myself accountable on many occasions. When there were times when I was having a hard time sticking to my nutrition protocols due to whatever factors (such as stress, etc.) I would commit to publicly sharing a picture of everything I would eat. I think you would be surprised at how many people are out there that will hold you accountable if you say you're are going to do this and do not.

The effect it has is twofold. First, I would think about things much more before I would eat them. "Do I want to hear these mother-fuckers make comments about this shit?" I would ask myself. Second, it got me thinking ahead of how to plan my meals out, so I would not feel tempted to have to post something that was not within my nutritional protocols.

To be honest, this is not a method that I suggest for people with food addictions. This is more for the person that just wants to have a little extra accountability in their nutrition. People with food addictions are highly prone to binge eating, and this particular method screams for it. Even if it does not happen the first day, you WILL end up substantially hungry at some point in time.

NUTRIENT TIMING

THIS SEEMS TO BE one of the best methods I was able to find that worked for me to manage my cravings throughout the day (I am not saying this is the only way or the best way, I am just saying, that for me, nutrient timing was very effective). I know, for me, about a half an hour after I eat a substantial amount of carbohydrates, I get very hungry a few hours after. What I did find is that if I just focused on eating mostly protein and fats throughout the day and then ate whatever carbs I was going to eat for my last meal, I wasn't fuckin hungry. I would do my normal fasting routine, where I would drink most of my fluids before lunch. Then I would have a huge serving of protein with some fats mixed in occasionally. Normally, some tuna from a can or tuna steaks. And while I was prepping that, I would eat my 2 ounces of walnuts for the day. This pound-size of protein and fats would satiate me without over filling my stomach until I was able to make it to my evening meal, which consisted of vegetables, some starches, and proteins.

All in all, a very effective way to control your calories (in my opinion, of course), but if you are the type of person that likes variety, you are kind of fucked as this simply does not provide that type of enjoyment. It is normally the same thing, or same type of thing, every single day.

PREPPING YOUR FOOD

I KNOW, I KNOW, you have heard this a 1,000 times before, but it really does make a difference. If you can manage to take just a few hours one day to prep some food for yourself for the week, you will be fuckin amazed at what can be accomplished. My food prep list normally looks like this:

Dice 1 Onion

Chop 5 zucchini

Dice 6 peppers

Prep 5 days of Protein Pancake Batter

Roast 3 pans of Broccoli

Dice 6 tomatoes

Thaw or clean 5 pounds of fish

Prepare 8 cups of beans

Crack and whisk 2 dozen eggs

All in all, it takes me about 45 minutes, and it leaves me capable of making veggie omelets, protein pancakes or waffles for my wife's breakfast, and throw together quick meals that take no longer to make than 15 minutes. This avoids me coming home and going straight to the fuckin cereal box. It also makes tracking my macros very easy. The thing is, again, not much variety as you end up eating the same types of meals all week. But guess what assholes: if you need to lose weight, especially a large amount, you are not going to be able to get that much variety. Food enjoyment is only for reward at this point.

DO NOT CHEAT... REWARD

PERSONALLY, I HATE THE term "cheat meal." These meals are basically meals outside a nutrition plan. The problem is that, from personal experience, and from coaching many overweight and obese people at this stage, cheating becomes very fucking easy to do. It is like that guy you know that cheats on his wife all the time. You would imagine that, at some point in time, he loved her enough to keep his dick in his pants and be faithful. Then, for whatever reason, he convinced himself it was ok to stick his dick in some other woman. Then, before you and the rest of your friends knew it, you were getting calls from his pissed off wife asking if he was with you four Sundays ago from 3 until 11 pm, and when you say, "I don't remember where I was yesterday," she screams into the phone, "I ALREADY KNOW YOU WEREN'T WITH HIM, I CHECKED YOUR FACEBOOK!" These are friends you do not need, because if they will cheat on their wife, they damn sure do not have enough self-control to not fuck you over, and that is the same principle with a cheat meal. The second a person who needs to lose a large amount of weight decides to cheat on their nutrition plan - the thing in their life that is trying to give them a good future -they will cheat more and more often until the nutrition plan is gone.

That is why I much prefer rewarding yourself with a planned meal. Every 10 pounds or so, the wife and I will plan a night out. The plan always has limits as it is a fucking plan. I will eat under my caloric plan by 200 calories for two days before the planned reward and for a day after, and then I will allow myself to eat 1,100 calories over on the day of the reward. The quick math on that is that I will eat over plan for the four-day period by only 500 calories or approximately 1/7th of a pound. I will still be in a very good caloric deficit for the week. My cravings will normally be very satisfied as I will even plan in a beer or two, and I won't feel like shit for cheating on the plan.

That is the difference between cheating on a diet and rewarding yourself according to your nutrition plan. One leaves you satisfied and with a sense of accomplishment, and the other makes you feel like a fuckin dirty loser.

So instead of cheating, try rewarding yourself, just make sure you fucking earn it.

TRACKING YOUR FOOD

I AM ALWAYS AMAZED at two things when it comes to suggesting to people that they start tracking their food and, thus, their nutrition. First, how resistant they are, and yet sure of themselves. They always seem to "know" about how many calories they eat but have never, ever, tracked their food, at all, let alone with an app. Second, how amazed, shocked... shit, *horrified* people are after they track their food for a week, and they realize how much they are actually eating.

See, that is a prerequisite for all my weight loss clients. Track your fucking food. If you cannot do that, I cannot fucking help you. If you will not take the time to push three things on your fucking phone to record the food you are about to eat or just ate then how in the fuck do you think you are going to hold yourself accountable to do all the other shit that is going to be required of you to lose the fuckin weight?

Oh, and they fuckin lie... god damn, do they lie. I have had 400-pound men send me their calorie totals every day for a week ranging from 1,600 to 1,800 calories a day with me telling them that they are doing a good job, and then weigh in day comes up, and they haven't lost a pound. FUCKING BULLSHIT!

If you look back to our boy Hemingway from the Math section of this book, it is easy to see that depending on the activity, they should be in at least a 2,000 to 2,500 calorie a day deficit (I am assuming 400-pound men will not be considered active let alone extremely active). This type of deficit works out to 4 to 5 pounds of weight loss in a week. It is 14,000 to 17,500 calories of deficit! You would lose fucking weight! It is just physics.

Recording your food is an amazing way to keep you on track (if you do not lie to yourself).

EAT FOR VOLUME

THIS IS A PRETTY easy concept, but is often the one people fuck up the most. If you are trying to lose weight, that normally means you are used to eating a larger amount of food than you should be (at least for the type of foods you are eating). If you are an obese person, there is a strong chance you are addicted to the feeling of having a full stomach, a certain type of food has an emotional connection for you, or both.

If you are a person that is overweight or obese and the main obstacle for you losing weight is that you hate the feeling of being hungry: EAT FOR FUCKING VOLUME.

I have had clients of mine, and have heard from others that specialize in fat loss, simply flat out fucking say they cannot survive on the amount of food they are told they need to eat. That 2,000, 2,500, hell, I have even gotten messages saying that eating 3,000 calories results in the person feeling they are starving and unable to stick to their nutritional protocols.

My response is always the same. There are an estimated 1,500 calories in ten fucking pounds of broccoli. Do you know how much volume 10 pounds of broccoli is?! If you can eat that in a day, you should enter food eating competitions, but until then, if you feel hungry, eat some high-volume foods that are not calorically dense.

Yes, it may be broccoli every day of your life forever, but at least you will keep your fucking legs and live to see your grandkids graduate high school.

Would you rather eat broccoli every single fucking day and enjoy the other aspects of your life much more, from walking, socializing, even having better sex? If you answered no to that and are an obese person, then I cannot help you. I wish you the best of luck in your half-assed effort to stop killing yourself via food and hope the double wide casket you are undoubtedly going to be buried in at a far too early age is nice.

The reality of the situation for an overweight or obese person is that they have OVER-enjoyed food. They need to understand that they have overindulged consistently for far too fucking long, and they are now hurting their very own lifespan. They do not need to enjoy every fucking meal like it was their last.

ONE FLAVORFUL MEAL A DAY

I HAVE OUTLINED IN this book that I adopted a pretty regular eating pattern around food intake when I was losing my weight. There are many reasons for that, from convenience to reliability, but most of all, it was helping me to not look like I had stuck an air pump up my ass making myself look like a balloon version of my younger self.

As I outlined earlier, I would have one of my two meals a day be a complete maintenance meal: fish and fats, normally with mustard. I know, weird, but you have just read me ranting for dozens of pages - you know I am weird. This allowed me to control my calories and have one meal a day that was more flavorful.

Our society has somehow adopted the idea that every little fucking thing needs to be enjoyable. Most of all, our food. Every meal is an indulgence. Think about the concept of pancakes - and yes, I fucking love them - but think about them. The word "cake" is in the fucking name, and yet, it is breakfast food. A decent percentage of people literally eat cake for fucking breakfast multiple days of the fucking week, and we wonder why there is not one state in the US that has an obesity rate below 20%... again, feel free to look it up if you do not want to take my opinion on it.

For lunch, sandwich places have convinced our society that eating nearly a whole loaf of fucking bread is somehow healthy for us. Think about the concept of how fucking ignorant to health and longevity this statement shows our society to be; that eating nearly a whole loaf of bread, often stuffed full of high sodium processed meats and high-fat sauces is somehow healthy for us. This is why the aliens do not need to invade; they are just going to wait for us to stupid ourselves out of existence.

Somehow, dinner comes with dessert almost every day of the fucking week. Do you have a birthday every day of the week? Did you get promoted every day of the week? NO, mother-fucker, you did not. You are just acting like every time you sit yourself down to eat there should be a fucking reward attached to it.

Truth be told, if you need to eat something enjoyable every day, start by trying to enjoy a normal sized portion of a tasty meal just once a fucking day. That is, of course, unless you are already in serious medical need of losing weight or they are going to start lopping off body parts. If that is the case, WAKE THE FUCK UP and realize you do not need rewarding at the dinner table. At this stage, the reward is you living past the next few years.

THE DRIVE-THROUGH WINDOW OF DEATH

WE LIVE IN A complete convenience society. It is one of the things, in my opinion, that is killing us. I am fucking amazed at how many people under the age of 30 barely know how to cook, and parents, that is your fucking fault by the way. So many people of the younger generation in our world today grew up eating multiple meals a week that were purchased through a drive-through window. These kids were set up for failure by their parents. And before too many of those parents that are reading this get ahead of themselves, I understand you may have been really fucking busy; I get it that you may have worked two jobs; I know that many of you did not intend to leave your child without one of the most necessary fucking life skills there is in being able to cook their own food, but that does not change the fact that if a person does not know how to cook, they are vastly more likely to be overweight.

Now that that is said, if you are a person who eats "fast food" (side note: the other day I went through a drive-through of a place with golden arches to get a fucking coffee and was asked to pull up to the "we don't have your order ready yet" line and wait, and it would be right out to me... how the fuck is that fast food?) on a regular basis and needs to lose weight (of which, most people who eat the shit that comes through a drive-through window do), please know that you cannot be taken seriously saying you are trying to lose weight. Losing weight is work. There is no way around it. Losing a life-altering amount of weight is staggeringly hard. It is not something that will be easy. If you are not willing to put in enough work and sacrifice by cooking all your own food, or at the very least, go to a restaurant that allows you to make healthier choices besides "do you want to supersize that," then you simply cannot be taken seriously as you are not truly fucking serious about it.

AVOID LYING TO YOURSELF

HAVING ENOUGH WILLPOWER TO lose any weight, let alone a large amount, is a delicate balance. Things such as lack of sleep, stress, family issues, boredom, and many other factors can definitely weaken the resolve of even the strongest of wills. One of the truly important lessons that I learned in losing my weight - do not fucking lie to yourself.

This is how people somehow convince themselves they are done losing weight before they have lost enough to be healthy: "I have already lost 50 pounds, and I feel great. I overestimated how much I needed to lose."

No mother-fucker, you did not. You are just sick of the sacrifice needed to lose weight. You realize that as you get smaller, you are going to be able to eat even less, and you still have to throw some extra activity into the mix to keep losing weight. The reality is that getting started for most people is one of the biggest challenges they face, once they start, the initial weight comes off relatively easy. It is not uncommon for an obese person of 350+ to lose 25 pounds of body WEIGHT in the first month of their transformation. This can have a horrible effect on the person as, in their mind, the calendar on how long it will take them to lose the 150+ pounds they need to lose just got much shorter. Most of them have told me that they thought that even though I warned them about it slowing down, they still managed to convince themselves that somehow it would stay at that pace.

They don't realize that a huge portion of that is water weight and food that was in their system. The nutritional intake of a person that eats their way to 350 pounds and up is staggering. Normally, the food is high fat, high sodium, and low fiber. This has an effect of making the body retain a lot of fluid, and a lot of shit. So basically, when the nutritional plan is put in place, it is normally moderate fat, low sodium, high fiber, and far less food. This has a shedding effect in the first few weeks that results in dramatic weight loss. They shed pounds and pounds of water weight, and the high fiber and less volume of food leave their digestive system emptier by a few pounds.

This can also have an effect of them not trusting the math. Even with a meticulous explanation to them that they cannot trust the scale in the first few weeks because the weight they will be shedding will not be all body fat… they lie to themselves and think that they can lose the same weight eating the same amount while having the same amount of activity until they are done. This is simply a fucking lie that, in my experience, 90% of overweight and obese people tell themselves. Honestly, it is probably one of the leading causes for why people quit at month 3 under the guise of "they have lost some weight." They do not see the same results in month 2 that they did in month 1, and all of a sudden come to the reality that they will actually have to fucking work harder and harder for it. AS THEY FUCKING SHOULD.

ACCEPT THAT IT IS YOUR FAULT

NOBODY FORCED YOU TO eat. Nobody forced you to sit on your ass. Even if you have been through some shit in your life - you have emotional baggage, had a bad childhood - nobody got you overweight or obese but you. Fucking accept it. It is important that you do. If you do not take ownership of it, you will not be able to rectify it. You will not be able to come to terms with the fact that because you are the one that put yourself in this position, you are the one that needs to get yourself out of it.

As I have said, now, and over, and over again, I specialize in weight loss for obese people. I have heard many stories about abusive childhoods, husbands and wives cheating, PTSD - you name it. And even though I probably seem like a complete asshole to most people reading this book (and even to many of my clients when they first start interacting with me), I have a hard time saying the things I need to say. You see, the world has coddled overweight people (in my opinion), and this is a huge fucking issue. This is why I openly state that things like the "Fat Acceptance Movement" are killing people (in my opinion). They make it either seem completely ok (I have even seen articles stating that you can be healthy at any size, which is simply not fucking true), all the way to the oldie but a goodie "you are not fat, you have fat."

No mother-fuckers… you are fat. If you do not want to be fat anymore, then make the life decisions necessary, apply effort and consistency to them, and change that shit. However, until you do so, you are fat, and you need to accept that.

YOU DO NOT HAVE FAT, YOU ARE FAT

THE SOONER YOU ACCEPT it, the sooner you can change it. However, by separating it from you, by making it seem detached, most people then tend to look at it as a thing that happened to them. Listen here, you mother-fucking assholes, I am bald. I do not have a bald head, I am fucking bald. It was not my choice, not one fucking thing I did could have changed it. All the men on both sides of my family are bald. There was no fucking hope. You know what I do with that. I fucking own it. I do not separate it from myself.

This is what fat people should do. They should fucking own it. Even if you have always been fat... you have always *been* fat. You have not always *had* fat.

Separating the fat into something you just *have* instead of it being who you are because of your actions relieves people of the responsibility of having it. It allows them to look at it as if someone else should take care of it for them, and that is just fucking horrible. It allows for fat people to act like a victim of their circumstances instead of the person that made the circumstances.

This type of mentality should be avoided for damn near all things in life, but especially for things in which your actions can directly affect your mortality.

ACCEPT FAT PEOPLE DIE YOUNG AND LIVE MISERABLY

THIS MAY JUST BE my opinion - just like this entire book. Being someone that was overweight, I can tell you that I was not fucking happy. Not at all. Yes, I did enjoy being stronger than I am now, but that was not nearly a big enough pay off for my belly getting in the way of tying my shoes. Lifting heavy weights did not stop me from getting pissed off every time I looked in a mirror and saw that round ass face. It was simply not worth it, and that was when there was at least some payoff. A payoff that most fat people do not enjoy.

Not being able to buy normal clothes sucks. Nothing about that felt good. I was amazed at how good I felt when I lost the weight. I knew I would feel better, but not that much better. Add to that, you just do not see many obese old people. Yes, there may be a few 300-pound people in their 70s, but not many.

Before I got back into fitness full-time, I did multi-unit nutritional management for skilled nursing, assisted living, etc. There were almost no obese people over the age of 70. Yes, there were some that were overweight - shit, they ate dessert at lunch and dinner - but there were almost no really large people above 300 pounds from my observation of 100s of facilities over the 12 years I did that for a living. I used to ask the doctors of the facilities about it, and they would all say the same thing. By the time a person hits their 60s, if they are obese, they start to accumulate multiple chronic diseases and disorders. They compound and aggravate one another until, eventually, it leads to the person's demise.

It is sad to think about, but it has always stuck with me. When I was around 250 and hit the age of 45, I was very aware that as I would go to these places for work, I wouldn't see people my size and, of course, I am not talking muscularly, I am just talking weight. It was one of the things that made it easy for me to decide to lose the weight.

SOME FINAL THOUGHTS AND TIPS

GET NEW FRIENDS

ONE OF THE HARDEST things for me when I was losing weight was being around the foods I loved to eat or drink. I fuckin missed beer so much! I was very lucky as my wife is a very healthy person and very into fitness, so the food we cooked in our house was, and always has been, very healthy and macro-friendly. She is into fitness and is a personal trainer, yoga instructor, and damn near everything else you can name, so I did have that portion of my life locked down to be healthy. Shit, most of my friends are either fitness professionals or very fit people themselves, so no transition was needed for me. I am not even stating that a change out of your entire social structure is absolutely necessary. What I am saying is that you may need to get some new friends.

The key things to look out for in cutting someone out of your life if you are trying to lose weight for any reason, but specifically to be healthy, are things like "you can skip the gym today, you've been going so much."

Yeah…either invite this person to workout with you, or lose their mother-fucking number.

If you are obese and someone says to you, "one (insert bad food choice item) won't kill you," tell them that you read a book from a middle-aged, bald mother-fucker that said it very well fucking could, and then have him call your doctor. Have your doctor explain the laundry list of dangers you IMMINENTLY face in your near future. If they still think it is ok for an obese person who obviously has an issue with self-regulating their food consumption to have just one under the guise that it won't kill them, give that mother-fucker the middle finger as you tell them to get the fuck away from you, permanently. That person is not your fucking friend to begin with if they would say something to you like that.

If you have a group of friends, or a friend that you indulge in lazy-ass behaviors with, it is possibly time to find a new group of people to hang with. If you and your friends get together once a week for bong hits, pizza, and video games, you may not be able to get to that next level on whatever time-suck of a game the group of you have been trying to become world champions at while you clog your arteries, give yourselves carpal tunnel, and exert absolutely no energy for 8-hour blocks of time.

If you are fat to the point that the doctor is warning you of the onset of chronic illnesses, such as heart disease or being pre-diabetic, then it is time for you to eliminate anyone in your life that would, in any way, stand in the way of you getting healthy. I know this may include some life-long friends, but are they worth dying for? Is someone that doesn't support you trying to live a happier, longer life worth keeping in your life. Just because you have had a friendship for a long time does not mean it is worth keeping, especially if the person gives such little of a fuck about you that they don't care about your health.

Keep an eye out for changes on the friends that you do keep. As you lose weight, you may trigger something in them that makes them feel bad about themselves and, thus, could make them, even unknowingly, try to sabotage your progress. I know this seems farfetched, but I can tell you that I have seen this happen. Shit, I have a client who divorced her hus-band because he refused to be supportive of her combating her food addiction. She lost close to 100 pounds and was feeling better about herself, and her husband started getting her trigger food back in their house. He was also obese but was still at the stage where he was going to "eat what he wanted because you only live once." After her 2nd backslide of 20 pounds due to binge eating her trigger food, she filed for divorce. She has now lost 160 pounds. I do not take credit for this, as she was only my client for 3 months after her divorce, but her story resonates with me about this subject all the time.

The whole point is that if anyone in your life is not good with you trying to be healthy, they are also not healthy for you. Just like the food that got you to be obese.

LOSE THE FAT CLOTHES

HOLDING ON TO "FAT clothes" is one of the most self-defeating thing people that are actively losing weight do.

For those of you that have never had to buy clothes that fit large sized people, they are more expensive than other clothes. I have recently heard some idiots (who are trying to make themselves feel better about being obese instead of accepting the thing) call it a "fat tax." For the record, that is one of the most idiotic fucking things I have ever heard of. Clothes for fat people use more raw materials by volume, normally need to be made with more structure to support the size at the seams, and they are often of a thicker fabric to prevent from tearing. They fucking should be more expensive. To put it into terms that these idiots understand… an extra-large calzone costs more than a small calzone because they have to use more of the ingredients to make it. It is fucking bigger and costs the restaurant more to make, so it is going to be more expensive. There, I hope that cleared that up for the "idiocy acceptance movement" people that will read this book just to slam it.

Since these clothes cost more money to produce, they are more expensive, and since the person that has to buy these clothes normally has a much higher food bill at the end of the month (notice I did not say grocery bill; you would be surprised how often restaurants, drive-thru windows, and delivery are the mainstays in the monthly food bill of an obese person), buying new clothes is a scary thought. However, the second clothes become too big for you to wear, throw those fucking things in the donation box and get them out of your house.

Do not hold on to fat clothes, as it gives you a safety net should you ever "need" them again. The only fucking way you will need them again is if you become that size again. If you keep them, you are pretty fucking much planning on it, so get rid of those fuckers as soon as possible. Then, if you slip and you feel the new smaller clothes that you spent money on getting tighter on you, it will be more of a wake-up call (instead of reaching into the closet and grabbing something "comfy" to wear. Comfy normally means bigger, mother-fuckers, or at least, it did for me). When faced with the choice of spending more money on more expensive clothes, it may be the thing you need to snap you back on to plan to finish losing the rest of the weight you wanted to or to at least get back to your goal weight.

EATING HEALTHY IS NOT MORE FUCKING EXPENSIVE

HOLY SHIT, THIS IS one of my trigger subjects. I hear people say all the time that eating "clean" or "healthy" is more expensive. This is one of the more fucking stupid things I hear often.

There is abso-fuckin-lutely no truth to this statement.

Yes, you can buy expensive rice in bulk; but you can also buy inexpensive rice in bulk. You can get bulk frozen vegetables at places like Costco that are incredibly inexpensive. Hell, if you look at the convenience, you can make your own fucking black coffee every damn day for about $.50 a large cup instead of buying that $4 cappuccino every day. Shit, if that is done 5 days a week for the work week, a person can save $17.50 and about 1,500 calories. That is a fucking winning situation. That is the cost of a commercial gym membership nowadays.

A meal at a drive-through window is almost always $10 or more; especially for an obese person. Whereas, at the local

Aldi's, you can get a pound of wild-caught frozen salmon for $3.50 and a 2-pound bag of organic frozen broccoli for $3. That is $3.50 less than the diabetes starter kit that a person picks up from the drive-through window that cost $10, and it will provide nearly all the protein, fiber, and many of the micronutrients a person needs every day while leaving you full as fuck, and that is splitting it over two meals.

The math simply does not add up, what-so-fucking-ever, that eating healthier is more expensive. What people normally mean by this is that it is less convenient for them as they need to prepare their food.

SOME AFTERTHOUGHTS AND COMMENTS

I WANTED TO THANK all of you for reading this. I personally know that I can be tough for many to take. My particular brand of satire and communication is not well received by everyone, and I do understand that. What I am hoping is that those of you who read this whole book see that I do not call people fat to hurt them. I do not ever intend to be directly insulting to people who are overweight or obese. I was one of them once, and I called myself fat damn near the entire time. To me, it is just a statement of fact. It is undeniable.

In life, you need to either accept the harsh realities of life, or you can try to avoid them. For people who have allowed themselves to gain so much weight that they are endangering their lives or, at the very least, shortening them, the choice to ignore the realities of their particular situation is a death sentence. It is a death sentence that comes with years of both physical and mental torture attached.

These are the reasons I am so blunt. These are the reasons I do not sugarcoat these words. The truth needs to sink in for people that are overweight and obese. They need to know that they can do something about it. They need to understand that while it may take a year to get to a healthy weight, they can at least fight for a life not encumbered by the self-induced prison that is their very own fat.

I gave up worrying about how the vast majority of people who need to lose enormous amounts of weight perceive me long agon. Frankly, I always go by the thought process that what people think of me is really none of my business. As long as I am trying my best to get through to at least one person… trigger that reality response for someone to say, "you know what, I am fucking fat, and I am going to die young if I don't change," I will feel accomplished in the writing of this book.

That means everything to me.

I like to strip away the bullshit of what the world tries to tell people to make them feel better about themselves and give them the harsh realities of what will actually make their lives healthier, happier, and better.

I truly hope that you found this book enjoyable, and if you are one of those people out there that don't need to lose weight to be healthier, it is a statistical anomaly that you would not know someone that does. So, while I know I already owe you a great deal of gratitude for buying and reading my first ever book, please do me this one last thing. Reach out to that person and tell them you are worried about them, and if they are willing to listen, you have something that may make them see what they can do about it….

AND THEN GIVE THEM YOUR COPY OF THIS BOOK BECAUSE YOU JUST MAY MAKE IT SO THEY WILL NOT BE THE REASON FOR SADNESS WHEN

THEIR CHILDREN OR LOVED ONES THINK ABOUT
THEM AFTER THEY ARE GONE FAR TOO YOUNG.

Thank you.

- Alan Roberts

REFERENCES

How to calculate Harris-Benedict Weight.

MALE CALCULATIONS HARRIS-BENEDICT WEIGHT

Pounds	Kgs	HB	Pounds	Kgs	HB
100	45.4	624	300	136.1	1871
110	49.9	686	310	140.6	1933
120	54.4	748	320	145.1	1996
130	59.0	811	330	149.7	2058
140	63.5	873	340	154.2	2121
150	68.0	936	350	158.8	2183
160	72.6	998	360	163.3	2245
170	77.1	1060	370	167.8	2308
180	81.6	1123	380	172.4	2370
190	86.2	1185	390	176.9	2432
200	90.7	1247	400	181.4	2495
210	95.3	1310	410	186.0	2557

220	99.8	1372	420	190.5	2619
230	104.3	1434	430	195.0	2682
240	108.9	1497	440	199.6	2744
250	113.4	1559	450	204.1	2807
260	117.9	1622	460	208.7	2869
270	122.5	1684	470	213.2	2931
280	127.0	1746	480	217.7	2994
290	131.5	1809	490	222.3	3056

MALE CALCULATIONS HARRIS-BENEDICT HEIGHTS

Inches	CM	HB	Inches	CM	HB
48	50.5	252.9	65	67.5	337.9
49	51.5	257.9	~ 66	68.5	342.9
50	52.5	262.9	67	69.5	347.9
51	53.5	267.9	68	70.5	352.9
52	54.5	272.9	69	71.5	357.9
53	55.5	277.9	70	72.5	362.9
54	56.5	282.9	71	73.5	367.9
55	57.5	287.9	72	74.5	372.9
56	58.5	292.9	73	75.5	377.9
57	59.5	297.9	74	76.5	382.9
58	60.5	302.9	75	77.5	387.9
59	61.5	307.9	76	78.5	392.9
60	62.5	312.9	77	79.5	397.9

61	63.5	317.9	78	80.5	402.9
62	64.5	322.9	79	81.5	407.9
63	65.5	327.9	80	82.5	412.9
64	66.5	332.9	81	83.5	418.0
65	67.5	337.9	82	84.5	423.0

MALE BG AGE

AGE	HB	AGE	HB	AGE	HB
10	67.6	35	236.4	60	405.3
11	74.3	36	243.2	61	412.1
12	81.1	37	249.9	62	418.8
13	87.8	38	256.7	63	425.6
14	94.6	39	263.4	64	432.3
15	101.3	40	270.2	65	439.1
16	108.1	41	277.0	66	445.8
17	114.8	42	283.7	67	452.6
18	121.6	43	290.5	68	459.3
19	128.3	44	297.2	69	466.1
20	135.1	45	304.0	70	472.9
21	141.9	46	310.7	71	479.6
22	148.6	47	317.5	72	486.4
23	155.4	48	324.2	73	493.1
24	162.1	49	331.0	74	499.9
25	168.9	50	337.8	75	506.6

26	175.6	51	344.5	76	513.4
27	182.4	52	351.3	77	520.1
28	189.1	53	358.0	78	526.9
29	195.9	54	364.8	79	533.6
30	202.7	55	371.5	80	540.4
31	209.4	56	378.3	81	547.2
32	216.2	57	385.0	82	553.9
33	222.9	58	391.8	83	560.7
34	229.7	59	398.5	84	567.4

FEMALE CALCULATIONS HARRIS-BENEDICT WEIGHT

Pounds	Kgs	HB	Pounds	Kgs	HB
100	45.4	434	300	136.1	1301
110	49.9	477	310	140.6	1345
120	54.4	521	320	145.1	1388
130	59.0	564	330	149.7	1431
140	63.5	607	340	154.2	1475
150	68.0	651	350	158.8	1518
160	72.6	694	360	163.3	1562
170	77.1	737	370	167.8	1605
180	81.6	781	380	172.4	1648
190	86.2	824	390	176.9	1692
200	90.7	868	400	181.4	1735
210	95.3	911	410	186.0	1778

220	99.8	954	420	190.5	1822
230	104.3	998	430	195.0	1865
240	108.9	1041	440	199.6	1909
250	113.4	1084	450	204.1	1952
260	117.9	1128	460	208.7	1995
270	122.5	1171	470	213.2	2039
280	127.0	1215	480	217.7	2082
290	131.5	1258	490	222.3	2125

FEMALE CALCULATIONS HARRIS-BENEDICT HEIGHTS

Inches	CM	HB	Inches	CM	HB
48	50.5	93.5	65	67.5	124.9
49	51.5	95.3	66	68.5	126.8
50	52.5	97.2	67	69.5	128.6
51	53.5	99.0	68	70.5	130.5
52	54.5	100.9	69	71.5	132.3
53	55.5	102.7	70	72.5	134.2
54	56.5	104.6	71	73.5	136.0
55	57.5	106.4	72	74.5	137.9
56	58.5	108.3	73	75.5	139.7
57	59.5	110.1	74	76.5	141.6
58	60.5	112.0	75	77.5	143.4
59	61.5	113.8	76	78.5	145.3
60	62.5	115.7	77	79.5	147.1

61	63.5	117.5	78	80.5	149.0
62	64.5	119.4	79	81.5	150.8
63	65.5	121.2	80	82.5	152.7
64	66.5	123.1	81	83.5	154.5
65	67.5	124.9	82	84.5	156.4

FEMALE HB AGE

AGE	HB	AGE	HB	AGE	HB
10	46.8	35	163.7	60	280.6
11	51.4	36	168.3	61	285.2
12	56.1	37	173.0	62	289.9
13	60.8	38	177.7	63	294.6
14	65.5	39	182.4	64	299.3
15	70.1	40	187.0	65	303.9
16	74.8	41	191.7	66	308.6
17	79.5	42	196.4	67	313.3
18	84.2	43	201.1	68	318.0
19	88.8	44	205.7	69	322.6
20	93.5	45	210.4	70	327.3
21	98.2	46	215.1	71	332.0
22	102.9	47	219.8	72	336.7
23	107.5	48	224.4	73	341.3
24	112.2	49	229.1	74	346.0
25	116.9	50	233.8	75	350.7

26	121.6	51	238.5	76	355.4
27	126.3	52	243.2	77	360.1
28	130.9	53	247.8	78	364.7
29	135.6	54	252.5	79	369.4
30	140.3	55	257.2	80	374.1
31	145.0	56	261.9	81	378.8
32	149.6	57	266.5	82	383.4
33	154.3	58	271.2	83	388.1
34	159.0	59	275.9	84	392.8

NEXT STEPS

Fitness is not owned by anyone. It is rented and the rent is due Every Damn Day.

For more tools and resources to help you to get to a healthy weight and stay there, visit us at:

EveryDamnDayFitness.net

ABOUT THE AUTHOR

ALAN ROBERTS IS THE founder of Every Damn Day Fitness and Co-Founder of the Damn Collective with his wife Crystal. Together, they have helped thousands of people increase the quality of their lives by coaching them to healthier habits, wisdom which they accrued through trial and error in their own lives. Originally from Pittsburgh, PA, Alan now resides in sunny, south west Florida.

Printed in Great Britain
by Amazon

38010100R00086